YOU'VE GOT THIS

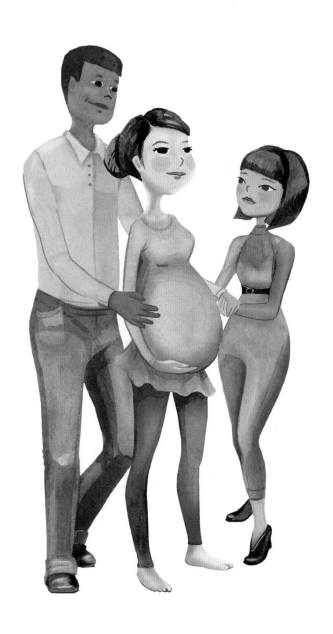

YOU'VE GOT THIS

Your Guide to Getting Comfortable with Labor

By Sara Lyon
Illustrations by Brittany Mash

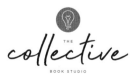

THE
collective
BOOK STUDIO

Library of Congress Cataloging-in-Publication Data available.

ISBN: 978-1-951412-21-0
Ebook ISBN: 978-1-951412-39-5
LCCN: 2020915632

Manufactured in China.

10 9 8 7 6 5 4 3 2 1

The Collective Book Studio
Oakland, California
www.thecollectivebook.studio

To BBC for the constant insipiration, and our kids who make me walk the talk. It's an honor to know you and love you. xxx

CONTENTS

"It is important to keep in mind that our bodies must work pretty well, or there wouldn't be so many humans on the planet."

Ina May Gaskin

INTRODUCTION

Welcome to *You've Got This!*

I'm Sara, the author of *You've Got This: Your Guide to Getting Comfortable with Labor,* and I'm deeply honored that you've chosen my book as part of your journey to parenthood.

Whether this is your first birth or your fifth, you're about to unearth some absolute gems in your reading. Why? Because I've been doing birth work all over the world since 2004, learning, teaching, and now collecting my favorite birth support techniques right here for you.

Through my work as a birth educator, doula, prenatal massage therapist, and author, I'm committed to helping families feel comfortable with pregnancy and the birth process, replacing any fear and insecurity with genuine confidence and excitement.

Educating birth support partners is just as important as educating pregnant mamas. Study after study shows that continuous, informed, familiar support is great for birth outcomes and for mama's satisfaction in labor. As the support partner, you might have some learning to do, but don't worry, you've got this!

To educate the support partner, I wrote *The Birth Deck: 50 Ways to Comfort a Woman in Labor.* The deck is a comprehensive collection of effective support techniques that are simply illustrated and explained with very few words, just enough to get the point across.

These flashcards for labor solve a problem I've seen over and over again: clients forgetting their birth education with the excitement of early labor. Since its publication in 2018, the deck has been adopted by expectant families, doulas, nurses, and midwives around the world, as well as by the state of California, which introduced them into more than 100 labor and delivery wards in an effort to reduce unnecessary caesarean procedures.

If *The Birth Deck* is simple and sweet, *You've Got This* is your guide to everything. In this book, I've included all the information from the deck plus much more, including expert tips, birth stories, activities, and fleshed-out instructions with detailed illustrations so you have a fuller and more functional view of comfort in labor.

What Is *You've Got This?*

You've Got This is a detailed guide to 50 tried-and-true comfort measures for childbirth. Written for mama and her support partner, *You've Got This* can be used solo or together as a team.

You've Got This is organized into four primary categories of techniques:

SUPPORT

The foundational tools that support the overall birth experience

MOVE

The most productive positions for labor

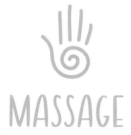

MASSAGE

The best massage techniques for comfort

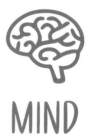

MIND

Scripts to encourage, calm, and emotionally support mama

At the end of this book, you will find the extra-juicy stuff:

Suggested techniques for approaching common labor challenges

Sequences for layering techniques

Your packing list for the birth center or hospital

A guide to finding the right doula

Resources for labor and postpartum

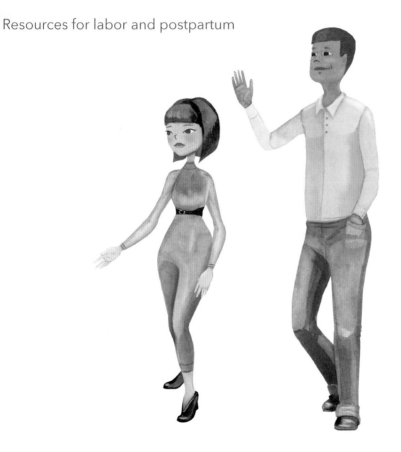

How to Use *You've Got This*

START

Read through *You've Got This* in order and then revisit mama's favorite comfort techniques (see LIKE, below) as you further prepare for labor. The techniques build on one another, so you'll have a well-rounded view of birth support by the end.

PRACTICE

Practice the SUPPORT, MOVE, MASSAGE, and MIND techniques, using the exercises in *You've Got This* to deepen your skills and build your confidence. Make this book your own—add notes and highlights wherever you want to so you remember the details as you practice.

LIKE

You'll find a blank heart on the bottom right corner of comfort technique pages. As you practice, note which pages you want to revisit in labor by filling in the hearts. This will provide easy reference for your support partner while you're focused on labor.

Keep an open mind: Techniques you didn't love before labor may bring you comfort once labor starts.

Example:

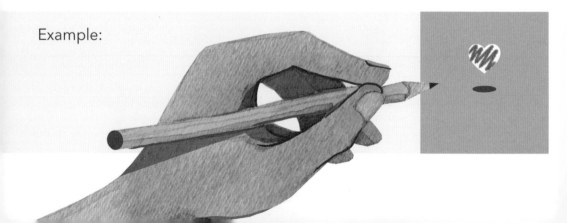

LAYER

Each technique can be used on its own, but I encourage you to layer the techniques for maximum effectiveness. When you layer techniques, you are addressing multiple sensory systems simultaneously, bringing ultimate comfort. You'll learn about mama's sensory systems when you read FOUNDATIONAL CONCEPTS in the coming pages.

Example:

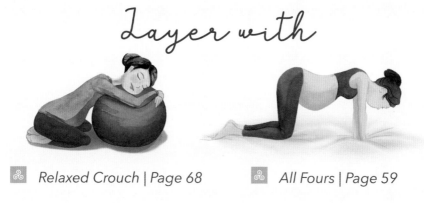

Layer with

🌀 *Relaxed Crouch | Page 68*   🌀 *All Fours | Page 59*

PREPARE

Use the SUPPORT section to pack your tool kit. Use the packing list and other resources at the end of the book to get ready for labor. If you have *The Birth Deck*, use mama's shaded hearts to organize your cards for easy use during labor, and don't forget to put the deck and *You've Got This* in your birth bag!

Foundational Concepts

PRIMAL BRAIN

Birth is all about the senses. How you perceive your surrounding environment during labor will have a physical impact on your birth experience and can even impact your birth outcomes. To understand this connection, we need to go back in time to our primal human days, before modern technology.

Humans were giving birth long before we lived in houses with locking doors and windows. We evolved to birth in the safety of nighttime, when predatory animals and other humans are usually sleeping. Accordingly, the hormones of labor heighten our senses, so we can take in all the safety information available in our environment through sight, smell, taste, touch, and sound.

Moreover, our pupils dilate so we're extra sensitive to light. Likewise, we're sensitive to smells, reactive to tastes, picky about how we're being touched, and hypersensitive to the sounds we're hearing.

In labor, we are using our super-senses to detect anything that could pose a threat to ourselves and this youngling we are about to release from the safety of our bodies into the world. Even though modern civilization poses very few threats compared to our primal days, we're still on high alert, and our senses continue to play a hugely important role in the course of our labors.

DISTRACTION

Luckily, you can use mama's superpowers to help her! Pain management scientists know that positive physical or psychological distractions can interrupt the pain sensory conduits to the brain. We want to bombard the body and mind with positive sensations, overriding uncomfortable signals to the brain.

This concept is known as Gate Control Theory and can be remembered like this: The brain wants to be happy. Give the brain a positive focus, and the brain will choose that focus over a negative one.

The comfort techniques in *You've Got This* will distract mama's brain from the intensity of contractions using thoughtful support, movement, massage, and mindfulness strategies.

LABOR'S ON AND OFF SWITCH: Oxytocin vs. Adrenaline

Oxytocin and adrenaline are hormones that can make or break the flow of a labor. They act as the on/off switch for labor. Oxytocin is released with trust, while adrenaline is released in response to fear. We will revisit this concept throughout *You've Got This*:

Trust = Oxytocin

ON

OFF

Fear = Adrenaline

Oxytocin initiates contractions and is only released when we feel safe and cared for. Oxytocin is stimulated by gentle touch, low lighting, positive mental imagery, soothing sounds, and an overall feeling of safety. Amazingly, oxytocin is also released by pain, which I explain in detail in THE CONTRACTION CYCLE, below.

Adrenaline shuts contractions down by signaling to the body that there is a threat to mama or baby. If the primal brain determines that it's not safe to release a vulnerable newborn into the world, labor stops while mama finds safety. Adrenaline is triggered by bright lights, encountering strangers, foreign smells, loud sounds, and general fear.

THE CONTRACTION CYCLE

Unlike almost all other experiences of pain, labor pain is not a result of injury; it's actually really productive.

Labor pain comes from the tightening of a big, strong, important muscle: the uterus. This muscular tightening is known as a contraction. Now is a great time to remind you that we want contractions; we need contractions. The contractions bring your baby into your arms!

Each wave-like contraction is triggered by oxytocin, our trust hormone. The contractions cause some amount of discomfort in early labor and build in intensity in active labor as you get closer to birth. Those sensations are a sign of power. Your body is powering your baby out into the world.

Brilliantly, oxytocin is released to soothe the muscular pain, and we have another contraction some minutes later in response. As the cycle evolves, the levels of all three rise consecutively in reaction to one another, and the labor builds in strength and frequency to the point of birth.

You've Got This will teach you how to use mama's senses to build her oxytocin and reduce her adrenaline, cultivating her trust and reducing her fear. Your calm presence, confident voice, and gentle hands are your greatest tools.

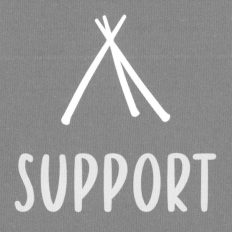

SUPPORT

Dear Support Partner,

Your role is simple: Bring your awareness solely to the needs of the laboring woman without distraction. If she's cold, make her warm; if she's working hard, give her water; if she's panting, help her breathe slowly.

Assuming some responsibility for birth preparation will increase mama's trust, thereby increasing oxytocin, the on-switch for labor. Try to predict her needs before she is even aware of them and plan for your own needs, like food, a change of clothing, and your own hydration.

The upcoming pages will guide you through thoughtfully packing your toolkit for birth. Page by page, you will learn how to use these effective support tools, many of which you probably already own. On page 140 you will find a simple packing list for your birth support toolkit.

Thorough support includes more than just objects and thoughtful gestures. Support includes the most foundational elements of a healthy labor: hydration and breathing. I'll teach you my foolproof breathing exercises for labor and the importance of a water bottle. Additionally, you will learn how to use the tone of mama's voice to reduce adrenaline, the oldest trick in the book.

Remember: *All you need is your hands, your heart, and few simple skills to provide hours of comfort in labor.*

xoxo Sara

Hydration

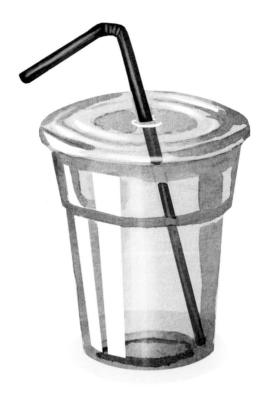

Would you run a marathon without water?

Of course not!

Hydration is the foundation of a healthy labor. Labor is a physical marathon and dehydration is a common and avoidable mistake.

As the support person, you are mama's pit crew, predicting her needs and arriving with the right tools to help.

Keep mama hydrated from the time labor starts until the end. Labor is hard work, and she is burning through fluids with every contraction.

It is your job to keep mama hydrated.

Fill a thermos or cup with one of the following:

- Water
- Half water, half juice
- Coconut water

Use a bendy straw so you can bring the water to her lips easily as labor becomes more intense..

Offer mama a sip between every other contraction.

Note: *If mama isn't allowed to drink fluids, offer her ice chips instead.*

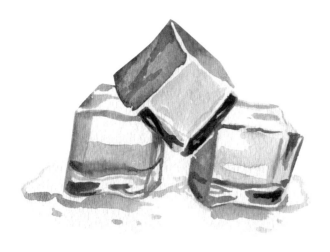

SET THE MOOD

It's worth your time to set up the labor and birth room for the optimal ambiance, first at home and then upon arrival at the hospital or birth center. Keep in mind that all of mama's senses are heightened, so be aware of the sensory inputs she's receiving through sight, smell, and sound.

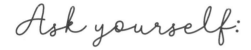

Ask yourself:

Is the lighting too bright?

Ask for it to be dimmed and turn on your electric candles.

Does it smell like hospital cleaning fluid?

Use your essential oils for aromatherapy.

Are the hospital monitors too loud?

Ask the medical team how you can turn the volume down.

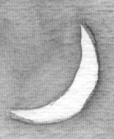

Sight

Most labors start at night, when oxytocin is naturally higher. We feel safer with the rest of the village at rest, knowing we can get on with the work of labor without distraction. Remember that the primal brain is constantly scanning for threats, and we can use senses to our advantage if we know just a few important facts:

In labor, mama's pupils will dilate, letting in extra light so she can see more clearly in the dark. Bright lights signal danger and will increase adrenaline, while dim lights or darkness will provide the safe cocoon she needs to labor in peace.

Lighting

Check that the lights are dimmed.

At home, draw the blinds and curtains. Keep lights low.

If someone has turned on brighter lights for an examination, soften them once they are no longer needed.

Bring electric candles to the hospital, as open flames are not allowed.

Smell

Use mama's sense of smell to mentally and emotionally transport her to a different time and place, relieving pain through distraction. Essential oils transform the birth atmosphere into a relaxing environment, encouraging effacement and dilation with their therapeutic qualities.

Diffuse these oils in mama's home when she is pregnant and relaxed so that she can access that calm feeling when she smells the oils in pregnancy:

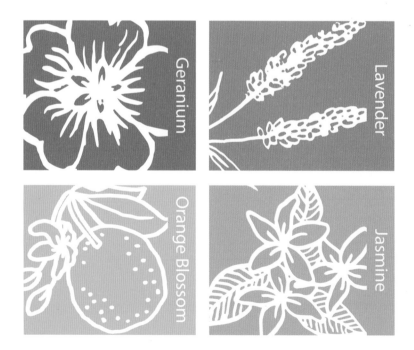

Geranium

Lavender

Orange Blossom

Jasmine

Aromatherapy

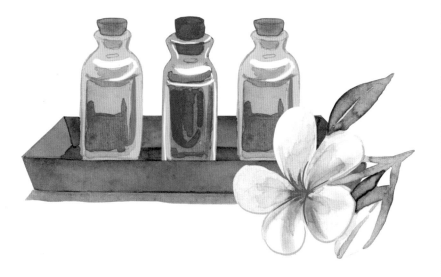

Bring aromatherapy oils to the birth place.

Place a drop or two of oil on a washcloth and place near mama's face.

Bring an electric diffuser to the birth place, if allowed.

Do not place oils directly on mama's or baby's skin.

The new sights, sounds, and smells of the hospital or birth center increase mama's adrenaline and reduce her oxytocin (see page 17). It's common for labor to slow down when first arriving as mama adjusts to her new environment. Remember:

Oxytocin

ON

OFF

Adrenaline

Challenge:

You've just arrived at the hospital and mama's labor slows down or stops.

Solution:

Getting to know your medical team and setting up the room according to the following tips can increase the labor-stimulating hormone oxytocin and reduce the labor-hindering hormone adrenaline quickly.

IT'S ALL IN THE DETAILS

Oxytocin is released with trust, and trust is built over time, through small gestures and sweet care. Be aware of mama's needs and try to fulfill them before she has to ask.

Ask yourself:

Are mama's lips chapped?

Lovingly apply lip balm for mama.

Is mama's mouth dry?

Offer her water and a mint.

Minty Breath

Nothing will get a birth support person kicked out of the labor room faster than bad breath, so keep both of you fresh by packing mama's favorite mints in your hospital bag. Don't forget to use them ;)

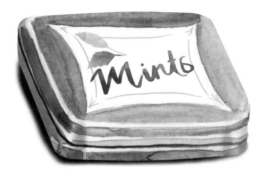

Bring mama's favorite mints and offer them to her occasionally for refreshment during all that heavy labor breathing.

Also, remember that mama's sense of smell is heightened, so be sure to use them yourself so that your breath is fresh!

favorite mints:

_____

Lip Balm

Hours of heavy breathing through contractions will leave both of you parched, so pack your hospital bag with two favorite lip balms, preferably in a stick for easy application. Bring the second one for backup in case you misplace the first.

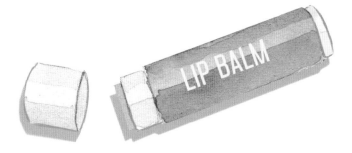

Bring mama's favorite lip balm and apply it for her when you notice her lips are getting dry.

favorite lip balm:

_____

Temperature Control

The hormones of labor flow in a symphony that's carefully calibrated for pain relief, opening the cervix, pushing, and then breastfeeding. These hormones also cause a variety of temperature changes throughout the course of a healthy, normal labor:

Early labor:

Comfortable

Active labor:

Hot and sweaty

Transition Labor:

Hot and cold flashes, sweating, and shivering

Pack a fan and washcloth in your hospital bag so you're prepared to support her needs as her hormones shift.

Fan

Fanning mama during labor will both cool her body and calm her mind.

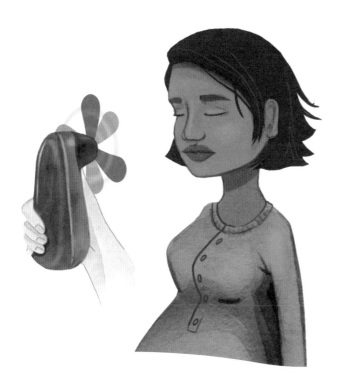

Create a comfortable breeze by fanning mama as she gets hot during and between contractions.

Use an electric handheld fan, a manual paper fan, or a magazine to fan her face and the back of her neck.

Washcloth & Blankets

It's normal for a woman in labor to feel hot and then cold, and then hot and then cold. Alternate between giving her blankets to warm up and using a cool washcloth to cool her down.

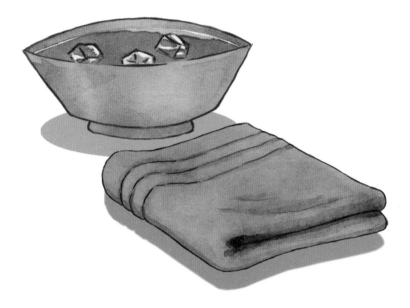

Place a cool, damp washcloth on mama's forehead and behind her neck if she is warm.

Keep a cup or bowl of ice water handy to dunk the washcloth once it becomes warm.

Use hot water to make a warm compress if mama is cold.

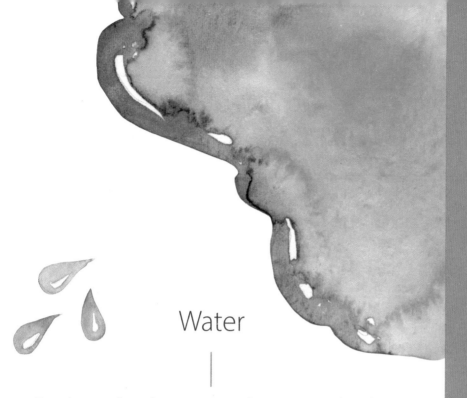

Water

Doulas and midwives consider water to be the epidural of natural comfort tools.

Gate Control Theory shows us that distraction will reduce our experience of pain, and there is no better distraction than a bath or shower.

The warm water touches so many nerve endings that the brain is bombarded with positive sensations, overriding the intensity of contractions.

Bath

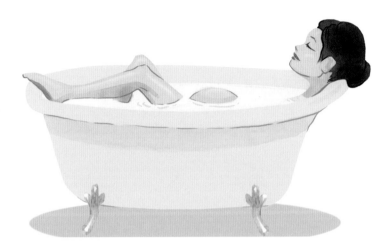

The immersive experience of a bath adds buoyancy, lightening the load of the baby and reducing the pressure on the pelvis.

Help her into the tub and get into it with her if she so desires.

Layer with

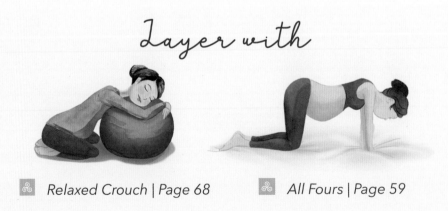

Relaxed Crouch | Page 68   *All Fours | Page 59*

Shower

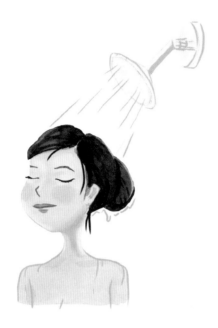

A shower's soothing pitter-patter distracts the body from contractions, allowing the brain's focus to shift instead to the warm drizzle, the skin's sensation.

Layer with

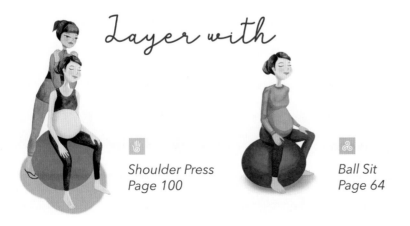

Shoulder Press
Page 100

Ball Sit
Page 64

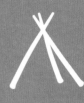

REST IS AS IMPORTANT AS WORK

|

The breaks in between contractions are crucial to maintaining stamina throughout labor; if mama is holding on to a contraction, she won't be able to rest adequately before the next one.

By relaxing her body and mind, mama will be able to quickly relax her uterus after every contraction.

Birth Story

"Breathing saved me! I was panting and getting light-headed, so one of the midwives started coaching me through the contractions, helping me breathe more slowly so that I was able to get full breaths. My contractions got stronger, but they didn't hurt as much, and my head stopped spinning. I'm so lucky that she'd seen so many labors and knew how to help me. It really changed the whole experience."

Olga V.

🌀 Home Birth   🕐 16 Hours   💊 No Meds

Breathing—It's Essential

If you feel like you're working out in labor, it's because *you are*.

Labor is aerobic exercise, and your uterus muscle requires oxygen to push a baby out. The uterus uses oxygen to contract its super-strong muscle fibers.

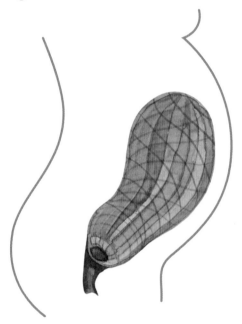

If you deprive your uterus of oxygen, it's not able to work efficiently, resulting in weak contractions and light-headedness.

While there are entire breathwork courses you can take to prepare for labor, we're going to focus on the foundational goals of breathing in labor: cleansing the body, focusing, and calming the mind.

Cleansing Breath

One

*As the contraction is beginning,
slowly say:*

Slowly take a big breath
deep into your belly, then
let it go completely out
of your mouth.

Two

As the contraction finishes, say:

Take a deep breath into
your belly, then breathe it
out completely. Let go of
the contraction.

Calm Breathing

Slowly and quietly say:

" Breathe slowly through your nose all the way down into your belly for 1, 2, 3, 4 seconds, and now breathe out through your mouth for 1, 2, 3, 4, 5." "

Breathe in:

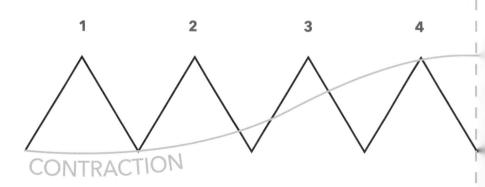

CONTRACTION

Breath Pattern

Fast, shallow breathing will increase the pain of a contraction, so encourage the laboring woman to slow her breathing by giving her something to focus on, like counting.

As she slows her breath, her mind will also relax so that she can better handle each contraction.

Breathe out:

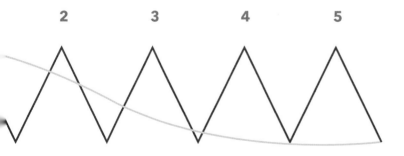

Groaning

Most women will naturally make a groaning, moaning or growling sound during contractions; it relaxes the jaw and cervix and distracts from the pain of the contraction, lulling mama into a calmer state through the vibrations of her deep vocalization.

As the old adage goes: "The sounds you made to get the baby in are the sounds you'll make to get the baby out!"

High-pitched vocalizations are produced by inadequate inhalations, a taught pelvic floor, tight jaw muscles, and a closed throat and tight mouth. These panicked sounds propel fear in a bad cycle.

Releasing the jaw reduces adrenaline as the jaw muscles relate to fear and self-defense; our teeth are our sharpest weapons.

Relaxing the mouth helps relax the cervix, as both are sphincter muscles.

Groaning produces bone conduction, the vibration traveling through your skeleton, releasing and relaxing the body and mind as it travels. Oxytocin is on the rise as your body relaxes and your mind settles.

By bringing the vocal tone down to a groan or a growl, the body and mind will follow. The baby needs to come down and out, through a relaxed cervix and a relaxed pelvic floor.

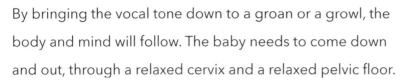

Challenge:

Mama is starting to pant, panic, or make high-pitched whimpers. This is a sign that her adrenaline is on the rise. Hearing her own voice at this pitch will trigger more adrenaline.

Solution:

Suggest that she make her noises deep and low-pitched so that she is groaning. Most importantly, groan with her, matching her volume and tone so she feels supported trying this technique.

Calmly say: "Bring your breath down to your belly and try groaning with me slowly with each exhalation. I will help by doing it with you: *Groooaaaaan*."

ACTIVITIES
This or That, Take 1

Women tend to birth how they live—but not always. It's important to learn about a variety of comfort techniques so you're able to use your entire toolkit throughout labor.

Look at the columns below and circle your preferences in each line. Then practice the techniques in this book and retake the test at the end of the book (page 125) to see if your preferences have changed.

Hot	Cold
Shower	Bath
Sitting	Standing
Deep massage	Light touch
Chatting	Silence
Upbeat music	Relaxing music
Lots of people around	Very few people around
Water	Fruit juice
Self-guided	Guided by support person

Visualization

Envision your optimal birthing environment.
What do you see?

_____

_____

_____

_____

_____

_____

_____

_____

_____

_____

_____

_____

_____

_____

SUPPORT

MOVE

Your baby is currently nestled in your abdomen like a key in a lock, with the head hopefully down in your pelvis. During labor, your baby's cranial bones will move closer together as your pelvic bones move apart, spreading just enough to allow the baby down and out.

Your body's transition to this moment has taken many months, nearly a year. Throughout your pregnancy, the hormone relaxin has been coursing through your body, softening your ligaments so they are more elastic.

Ligaments are the tight bands connecting our bones to one another, creating joints that move. Relaxin increases the flexibility of these tight bands for the express purpose of allowing the baby to fit out of your pelvis during birth.

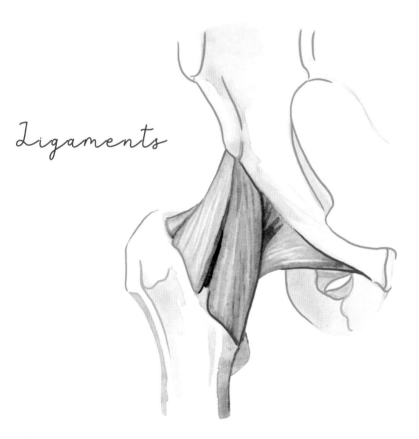

Ligaments

As your labor progresses, moving your pelvis is critical. Your movement allows the baby to navigate the bony prominences of your pelvis to find the best position for birth. The baby's position is critical to your birth experience, impacting the length and sensations of your labor, the efficiency of your contractions, and the effort required during pushing.

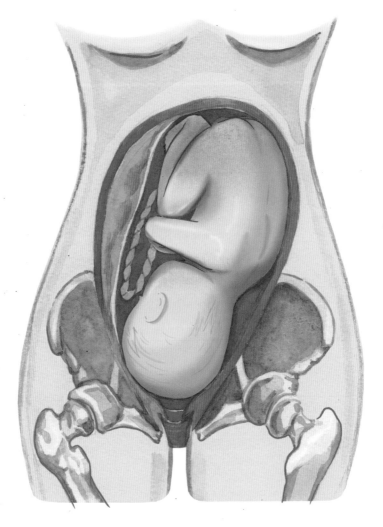

Share and explore the Move section with your support partner. Practice at home, finding the best positions for your body and the most useful props. Become familiar with new positions and be sure to note your favorites. Remember: You can't always predict what you will want or need in labor, but you can try!

In the Resources section, you will find the details for Spinning Babies (page 126). I highly recommend you take a look at their information during pregnancy so you can help your baby into the best position for birth.

Birth Story

"Labor started really slowly, and it took 12 hours for my contractions to get strong. Once active labor started, all I wanted to do was sway my hips, rest my head on my husband's shoulder, and groan through every contraction, like we were slow dancing except there was no music on. I did this all over the labor and delivery ward, in the hallways, and the stairwell. And when labor got really intense and we were just a couple hours away from our daughter's actual birth, I would hang on his neck with more of my weight and let my hips relax during the big contractions."

Jamie B.

Hospital   18 Hours   IV Meds

Slow Dance

Mama's body needs to move so that the baby can move down in her pelvis. Upright positions, combined with movement, will help labor progress, bringing you closer to birth.

Suggest that mama hug you while standing, wrapping her arms around your neck.

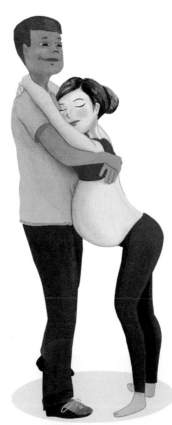

Begin to sway, or dance slowly, helping her move her hips.

During contractions, allow mama to hang on your neck with her arms so that she can move through the contraction.

Layer with

Any and all Mind techniques (pages 102–123), speaking quietly to her as you sway

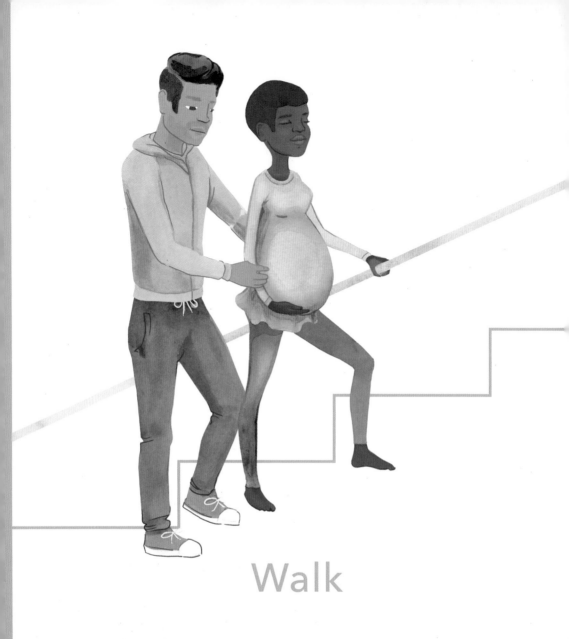

Walk

Walking the neighborhood, the halls, and the stairs can help dilation and move the baby into a good position for birth.

Suggest that mama walk, walk, walk!

Pause for contractions and physically support her if needed.

Challenge:

Mama refuses to move and she doesn't have an epidural. She's been in the same position for a long time and contractions have slowed down. It might be time for her to try some movement to help her labor progress.

Solution:

Strongly, lovingly suggest that she brush her teeth—minty freshness is motivating. Voila! She's up, the baby's weight is down on her cervix, and she's having stronger contractions, a good sign.

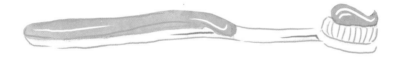

Brush Teeth

It can be meditative, relaxing, and refreshing to do something as familiar as brushing teeth.

Help mama move over to the sink, pausing for contractions, and put the toothpaste on her brush for her.

Now that you have mama up and moving, you can suggest other techniques from the MOVE section to help labor progress.

MOVE

FORWARD LEANING

Forward-leaning positions are the bread and butter of labor movement—they provide the perfect base for most massage techniques and help the baby move into optimal positioning for birth.

Leaning forward naturally relieves pain in the hips and lower back as the baby's weight moves off the tailbone and spine. Your hanging belly becomes a hammock, giving the baby more room to move for their comfort and yours.

All Fours

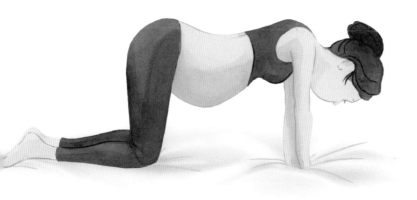

This position relieves pain in the hips, lower back and belly.

Suggest that mama get on all fours on a thick yoga mat on the ground or a bed to protect her knees and wrists.

Layer With:

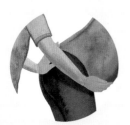

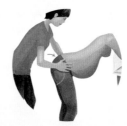

Back & Belly Hold
Page 83

Double Hip Squeeze
Page 84

Lean on Counter

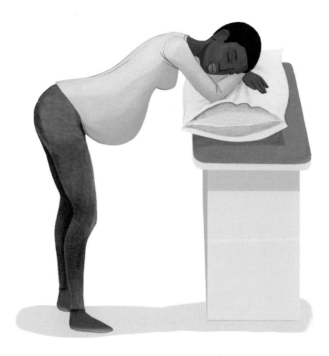

This position will relieve pressure in the hips and pain in the lower back.

Suggest that laboring mama lean forward onto a counter, baby-changing table, or high bed (hospital beds can be adjusted) while standing.

She should be supporting her upper-body weight.

Add appropriate MASSAGE techniques while she's in this position.

ACTIVITY
Mix & Match

Pick a technique from each category to combine with Lean on Counter:

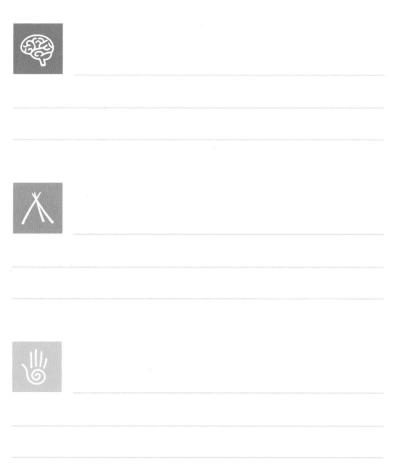

THE BIRTH BALL

Meet your new best friend for pregnancy,

birth, and baby-calming.

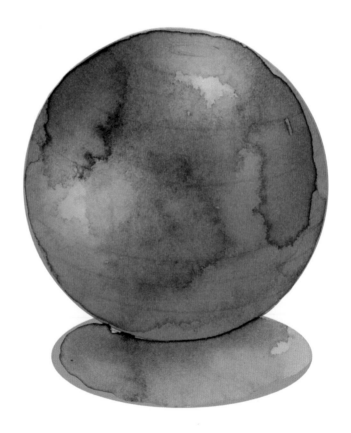

The birth ball is a foundational tool for movement in labor. The malleable surface of the ball allows your pelvic bones to move naturally so the baby can move through and out for birth. A flat surface, like a chair or mattress, won't allow the same movement.

Over the next few pages, you will learn the most effective positions and sequences using the birth ball. Practice them at home prior to labor so they're second nature when it's time for action.

Expert Tip: Bring your own ball to the hospital so you're guaranteed a clean, familiar prop—they won't think you're crazy, I promise.

While some hospitals and birth centers have balls for you to use in the labor and delivery ward, there's no guarantee they will be the most comfortable size (commonly 65cm), and they are often deflated.

MOVE

Ball Sit

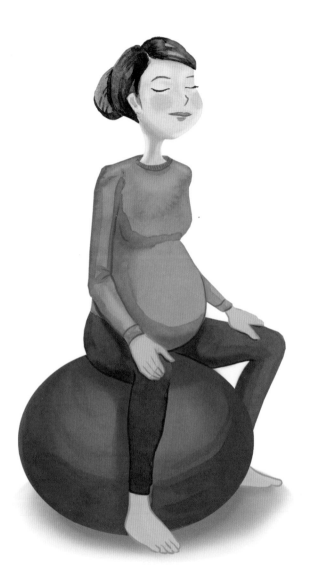

Let gravity do its thing in this upright seated position.

Try rotating the pelvis in a circular motion to help the baby move into the most comfortable position, relieving mama's back pain.

This pelvic motion combined with gravity will help the baby descend, bringing mama closer to birth.

Suggest that she sit on a birth ball and rotate the pelvis with the movement of the ball under her.

Add appropriate Massage techniques: *Shoulder Press (page 100), Arm Stroke (page 89), and Third Eye Stroke (page 92).*

Expert Tip: Your birth ball is also your ultimate baby soother/back saver—the gentle bounce of the ball will lull your infant into a gentle rhythm while you give your back a break from standing. Sit on your ball with your baby cradled securely in your arms and gently bounce up and down. Note that in the first 6 weeks, this is a job for the support person, not for the recovering mama.

MOVE

Ball & Bed

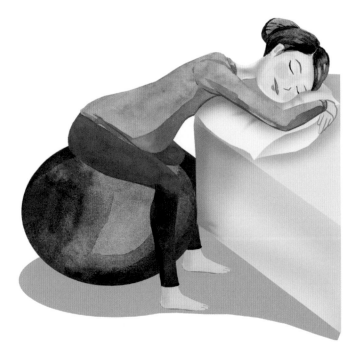

Remember: Rest is as important as work. When mama needs rest between contractions, she should relax her upper body on to the bed and pillows. In this position, she can catch her breath, let her abdominal muscles and uterus relax, and calm her mind.

This position also allows mama to be active during a contraction by rising onto her forearms on the bed while she focuses on breathing.

Add pillows if the bed is too low for her comfort—mama's belly should not be pressing on the ball between her legs.

ACTIVITY
Pick & Choose

Ball & Bed is the perfect position for layering massage techniques. Mama, list your favorites here:

Relaxed Crouch

Try this combination of *Relaxed Crouch* and *Lean on Ball* through a contraction. Add Ball & Forearms during active labor.

①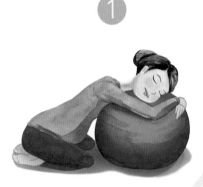

②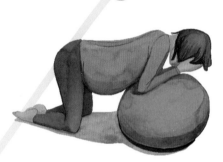

Relaxed Crouch

In between contractions: Mama will sit on the floor with legs folded under her, hips on heels. She will lean forward so that her entire upper body is supported by pillows or the birth ball.

Ball & Forearms

At the height of the contraction: Suggest that mama place her forearms on the ball and her head in her hands so that she can be even more active in the contraction.

Lean on Ball

This sequence positions allow mama to be active and focused at the height of tension, and relaxed in between.

③

④

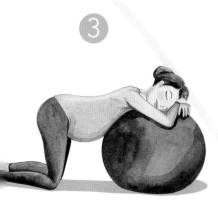

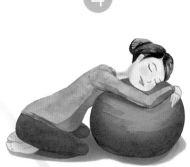

Lean on Ball

As the contraction strengthens: Suggest that mama lean over the birth ball, a sofa, or a large stack of pillows with her knees on the ground, possibly wagging her hips back and forth to relieve pressure.

Relaxed Crouch

Mama will sit back down on the floor with legs folded under her, hips on heels. She will lean forward so that her entire upper body is supported by pillows or the birth ball. Suggest that she take a *Cleansing Breath* (page 43).

Side Lying

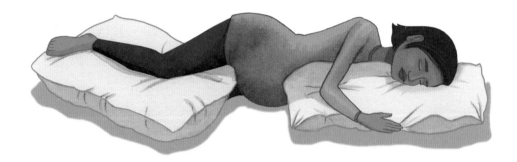

The side-lying position is helpful throughout labor, from early labor to the pushing stages, and is the preferred position if an epidural has been administered.

Layer with

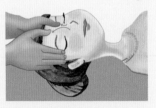

🖐 *Third Eye Stroke | Page 92*

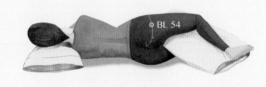

🖐 *Bum Press | Page 97*

If mama is fatigued and needs to lie down, or if she has had pain medication that requires her to recline, suggest that she lie on her side with pillows between her arms, with bent knees and ankles (a body/pregnancy cushion works perfectly).

Add more pillows between her knees if her hips are sore in this position.

Remember that the baby needs mama's movement to move down through the pelvis, so every 20 minutes help mama switch sides with your help.

Add Massage techniques to make this position ultra-comfortable, like *Third Eye Stroke* (page 92), *Bum Press* (page 97), *Arm Stroke* (page 89), *Ankle Press* (page 99).

Layer with

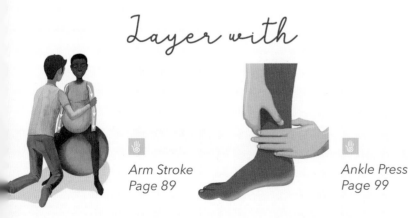

Arm Stroke
Page 89

Ankle Press
Page 99

Toilet Sit

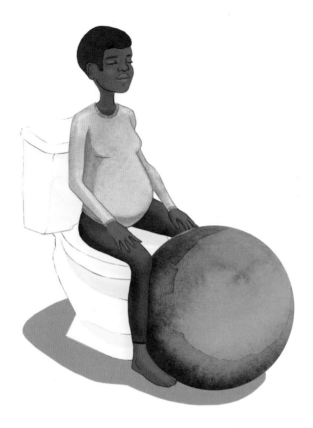

Suggest that mama sit on the toilet.

She can lean forward, supporting her upper body with her forearms on her thighs.

Variation: Place the birth ball in front of her and you can sit on it to support her physically and use Mind techniques to soothe her. Alternatively, she can lean onto the ball for support between contractions.

Sh*t Happens

Mama,

The bathroom is a place we associate with letting go, which explains why the toilet is often the most comfortable place to labor. It's a familiar place to relax your bottom and eventually push.

Your bowels will likely be crampy at the onset of labor. The good news is, bowel movements stimulate uterine contractions and make room for the baby to move down.

If you notice that you're feeling nervous about the pressure in your bottom as labor progresses toward pushing, have a seat on the toilet again and see if it allows you to relax your pelvic floor so you can start to bring the baby down farther into your pelvis and closer to birth. Sitting on the toilet may help you let the pressure move through you instead of resisting it.

Support Partner,

Your job is to help mama feel comfortable with the variety of intense sensations she's experiencing throughout labor, and bowel pressure is just another one of those! Guide her to the bathroom if you see that she's holding back or feeling self-conscious about the way her body is responding to labor.

MOVE

Squat

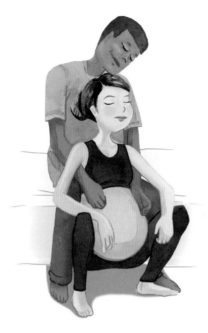

Squatting uses gravity and mama's body mechanics to encourage the baby to descend, promote cervical dilation, and assist with pushing.

Make sure mama is totally supported so she can put all her energy into the contraction.

Sit in a chair and spread your legs wide apart.

Suggest that mama stand between your legs, facing away from you.

Have her squat between your legs while you are sitting comfortably, using your thighs for underarm support.

Support her weight entirely with your legs under her arms.

Birth Story

"I was so excited to find out how dilated I was, and when the OB checked, I was close to fully dilated but not quite close enough to start pushing. I was disappointed to still have 2 centimeters left—it felt like 10 centimeters to me at that moment. But we found the Squat card in *The Birth Deck* and tried it. It only took 15 minutes, and it was like my cervix just scooted out of the way, and suddenly it was all happening: My water broke, I immediately felt the urge to push, and 30 minutes later our son was in my arms!"

Marcella L.

 Hospital   27 Hours   Nitrous Gas

MOVE

"You can't stop the waves, but you can learn to surf."

Jon Kabat-Zinn

ACTIVITY
Overcoming Challenge

Think about a time when you faced and overcame a great challenge like a sudden life change, a difficult task, a broken relationship, or a work disappointment. What emotions, feelings, and traits did you use to overcome this challenge?

MOVE

MASSAGE

Unsurprisingly, massage is the most popular category of support techniques. Always welcome, massage is fun to practice and easy to master if you're willing to take feedback from mama.

To understand why massage is so effective for pain relief, consider the way the body communicates with the brain. Our nerves are like electrical wires connecting our bodies to our brains. These wires transmit physical sensations from the internal and peripheral body that are then interpreted for meaning by the brain: Pain! Pleasure! Hot! Cold! Our emotional reactions follow this messaging.

There are billions of nerves ending at the surface of the skin, making touch a fantastic way to introduce positive, distracting sensations during labor. Massage can be as simple as a gentle hand on the lower back or more intentional, like acupressure. Your hands can provide hours of support, especially in moments when mama wants silence but still needs comfort.

Before learning specific massage techniques, it's helpful to understand the simple differences between massage styles. In the following pages, you will first learn about three different massage categories and their best use throughout labor. Finally, you will get instruction on my 13 favorite massage techniques for labor.

Expert tips:

Don't overthink it! Your conscious touch is the most important element, not your technique.

Don't take it personally! Keep yourself open to mama's feedback.

Keep your hands steady and slow! Don't move too fast.

Massage Categories

Massage styles, techniques, and their best uses.

Static

When: *During* contractions in active labor and the transition to pushing

Why: Soothes the intensity of contractions by providing counter pressure that makes women feel physically held and well supported in labor. Her mind is focused on riding the waves of contractions.

Dynamic

When: *During* contractions in early labor. *Between* contractions in active labor and the transition to pushing.

Why: Distracts from the increasing intensity of early labor contractions but can be annoying during the big active contractions that require mama's undivided focus; instead, try Static techniques during active labor.

Acupressure

When: Any time after 38 weeks. *During* contractions in early labor. *Between* contractions in active labor and the transition to pushing.

Why: Traditional Chinese medicine acupressure points have been used for centuries to relieve pain and help labor progress. These techniques are deeply therapeutic, impacting the nervous system directly and encouraging dilation and contraction.

Leg Squeeze

Back & Belly Hold

Double Hip Squeeze

Tailbone Press

Arm Stroke

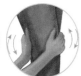

Shake the Tree

Third Eye Stroke

Belly Dance

Lower Back Stroke

Bum Press

Ankle Press

Foot Press

Shoulder Press

Leg Squeeze

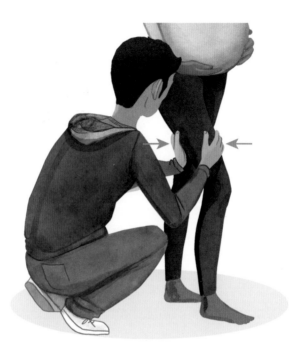

Squeezing the leg invites fresh circulation and relief to sore leg muscles after hours of labor.

Squeeze one leg with both of your hands, moving down the leg from the upper thigh to the foot.

Simultaneously compress the inner and outer sides of the thigh. Skip the knee joint. Compress the back of the calf, the sole of the foot, and the tips of the toes.

Repeat on the other leg.

Back & Belly Hold

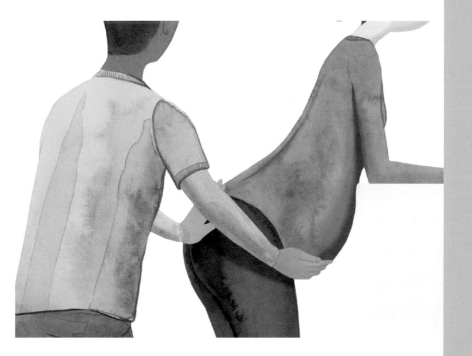

Use the warmth and comfort of your hands to bring relief to mama's sore lower back and her contracting belly with this deeply supportive static hold. This technique also offers a sweet way to connect with the baby during labor.

Stand behind mama while she leans forward, resting her upper-body weight on a bed, ball, counter, or wall.

Hold her tailbone confidently with one hand and hold her lower belly with your other hand. Do not rub her belly, just hold both hands still.

Double Hip Squeeze

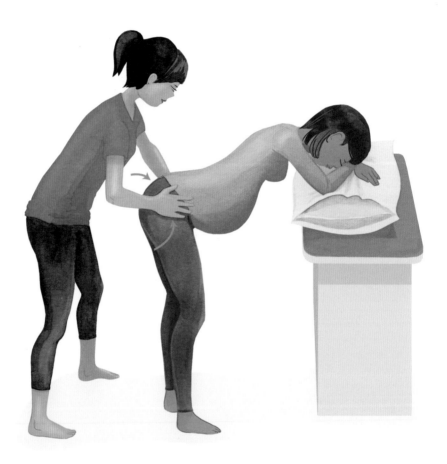

As the baby moves down in the pelvis, it's normal for women to experience pain and pressure in the hips. The *Double Hip Squeeze* relieves pain and brings comfort through counterpressure.

84

Mama is on her hands and knees, or leaning forward on a countertop, birth ball, or bed, or against a wall.

Place your palms on the sides of mama's hips.

Lean forward so that your chest is above her tailbone; this will give you maximum power to squeeze. You should feel the fleshy part of the hips (not the glutes) under your palms—nothing bony. The farther forward you lean, the more power you will have to push your palms into her hips.

Now, press your palms together until mama is feeling relief. Hold steady during contractions and release between them.

Expert Tip: When in doubt, Double Hip Squeeze.

Tailbone Press

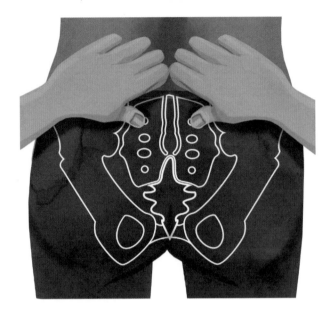

As the baby's head moves down in the pelvis, it presses nerves on the inside of the tailbone, causing pain. The *Tailbone Press* significantly relieves this pain through massage.

Press points on her tailbone with your thumbs.

Have mama lean forward onto a countertop or bed.

Starting at the top of the tailbone, hold the pressure firmly to mama's comfort level, using your thumbs and elbows; hold for five seconds, then move down an inch and repeat until you have pressed four points down the tailbone. Repeat as desired.

Expert Tip: Combine the *Tailbone Press* with the MOVE technique All Fours to set up the perfect positioning for the fastest results.

Why? Nerves running from the uterus up the spine to the brain transmit the pain signal from contractions. These nerves are easiest to access when the pelvis is rotated forward. Pressing on the tailbone relieves discomfort by interrupting the pain signal in those nerves.

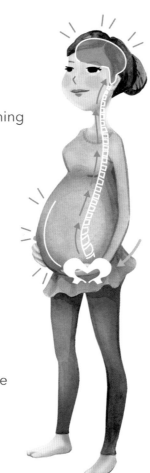

Layer With:

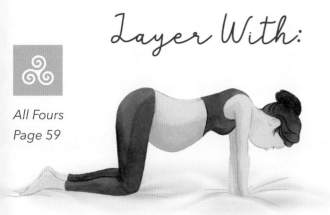

*All Fours
Page 59*

Birth Story

"My girlfriend was so anxious about labor; I was calming her down in the months leading up to our due date. I ended up getting induced and, luckily, the induction was pretty smooth, but the contractions were really intense really quickly. Suddenly I got nervous. My girlfriend came up to me and slowly brushed my arms over and over again; it was so calming. She kissed my forehead and said, 'You are so strong, and I am so excited to meet our baby; thank you for doing this for us.' It felt like the beginning of the rest of our lives."

Christy V.

 Hospital   20 Hours   Epidural

Arm Stroke

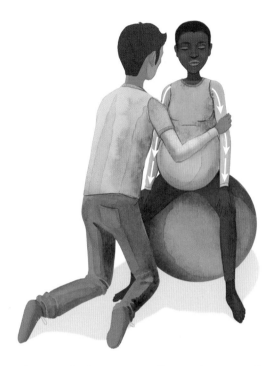

This grounding technique uses distraction to relieve pain by moving mama's focus from the contraction to the comforting arm stroke. If you see her shoulders moving up toward her ears, or her fists clenching, or if you hear her voice rising to a high pitch, use your hands to simply bring her attention back down into her body and into the room.

Stroke down mama's arms from her shoulders to her hands.

Use firm and steady pressure for the stroke.

Do not break contact, and move slowly so your touch is very calming.

Shake the Tree

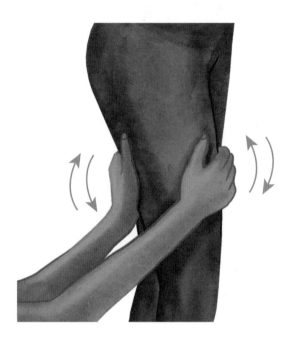

Jostling the muscles of the legs between contractions will relieve sore legs and hips.

Between contractions, shake one thigh at a time while mama is leaning forward onto a countertop or bed, or against a wall.

Wrap both hands around one thigh.

Rotate your hands clockwise first and then counterclockwise so you are moving the muscles of the thigh right and left. Repeat this rotation 5 times.

Switch thighs and repeat.

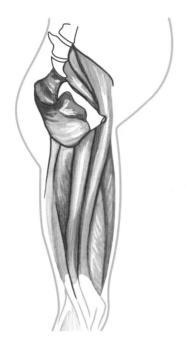

Expert Tip: Use this technique when mama's lower back, legs, or hips are sore.

The upper leg muscles start at the pelvis. These are the same bones that make the lower back and hips. When you rotate the muscles back and forth vigorously, you are loosening the entire hip and lower back area along with the thighs.

Additionally, it's deeply distracting to have so much movement during or between contractions literally shaking things up.

Third Eye Stroke

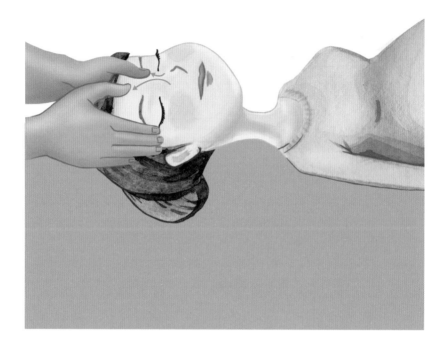

This motion should be restful and calming to help mama's nervous system settle down.

Slowly and sweetly stroke the area between mama's eyes up toward her forehead with light to medium pressure.

Repeat slowly 5 to 10 times between contractions.

This is a perfect opportunity to use some of the MIND techniques (pages 102–123) simultaneously.

Belly Dance

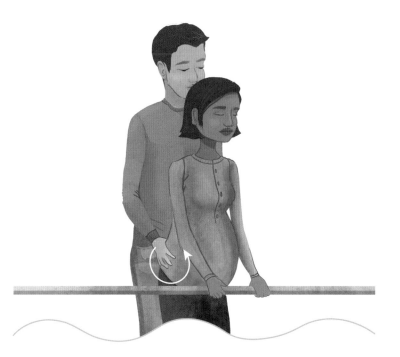

Mama's body needs to move to help the baby descend. This *Belly Dance* motion can help relieve pressure and pain through the lower back and pelvis during and between contractions.

Mama is standing straight up or leaning forward onto a countertop or bed, or against a wall.

Guide mama to rotate her hips at a slow to moderate pace by holding her hips and moving them in a rotating flow like she's a belly dancer.

Lower Back Stroke

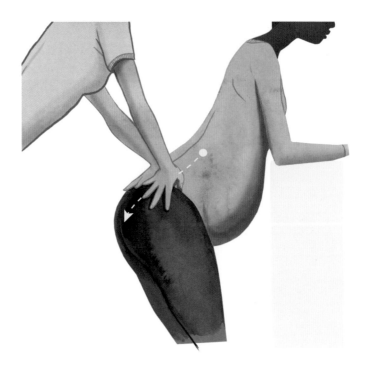

Rub mama's lower back, slowly moving toward her tailbone with smooth, firm strokes.

Repeat 10 to 30 times depending on mama's desire.

You can use lotion or oil if mama is undressed and not in water, but it's not necessary.

Expert Tip: Use your full hand with the focus of the pressure on the heel of your hand.

This technique will bring comfort and pain relief during and between contractions, but it's particularly soothing in between challenging active labor contractions. The firm pressure of the hands gives solid counterpressure while the friction on the skin is pleasantly distracting.

Try this sequence as mama flows through a contraction:

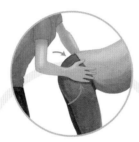

Double Hip Squeeze
page 84

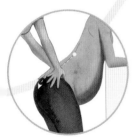

Lower Back Stroke

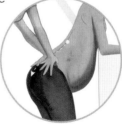

Lower Back Stroke

Cleansing Breath
page 43

Cleansing Breath

Birth Story

"So, I'll be honest, a lot of the acupressure didn't feel that amazing, not like the rest of the massage techniques my doula used that were immediately relieving. Wisely, our doula explained that the points were sort of medicinal. They are used to help with something specific, not just to relax the body and mind generally, although apparently, they do that too. The acupressure massage felt sharp, and I had to breathe through the pressure for some of them, but it was worth it because they helped my labor move along when it had stalled for long enough that my OB was talking about using Pitocin to get things moving again. After 20 minutes of deep pressure on my shoulder, ankle, and hips, labor had picked up again. I had to deepen my breathing to cope with the pressure of the massage points, and I think that relaxed the rest of my body, too, because fighting the pressure made it more uncomfortable than just surrendering to it, much like the contractions."

Shari S.

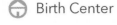 Birth Center   18 Hours   No Meds

Bum Press

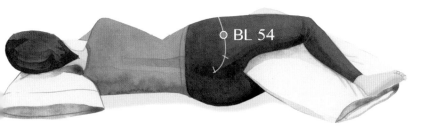

BL 54

Do not practice this point until 38 weeks or later.

This acupressure point relieves pelvic pain and relaxes the hips and lower back, helping release the pelvic muscles and joints so that the baby can descend.

Press the Bladder 54 acupressure point in the middle of mama's gluteal muscle with your elbow.

Start with very light pressure and adjust pressure as requested by the laboring mama.

Foot Press

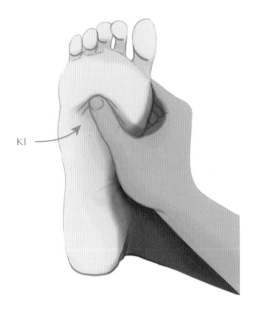

KI

 Do not practice this point until 38 weeks or later.

This point draws the energy down toward the feet, helping the baby descend and relieving the pain of contractions.

Press the Kidney 1 point on the bottom of mama's feet with your thumbs.

Mama can be side-lying or on her hands and knees.

Find the soft point just under the ball of her foot and press firmly with your thumb. Hold this for 15 seconds.

Ankle Press

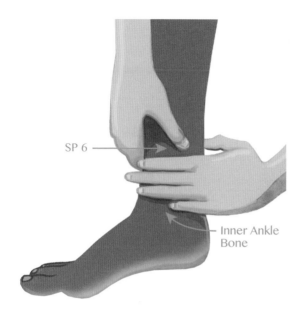

SP 6

Inner Ankle Bone

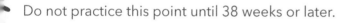

Do not practice this point until 38 weeks or later.

This powerful point helps the cervix relax and open.

Press the Spleen 6 point on the inside of mama's ankle with your thumb.

Press straight against the bone with medium pressure and hold for 15 seconds during a contraction. It's normal for this point to be sensitive.

Expert Tip: Spleen 6 can be particularly uncomfortable when pressure is applied, but that pinching feeling is crucial to activate the point.

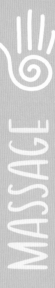

Shoulder Press

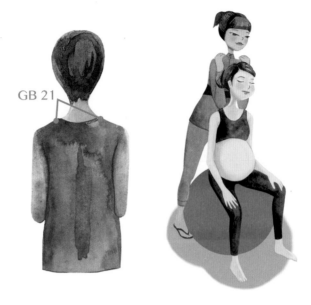

GB 21

Do not practice this point until 38 weeks or later.

The English translation of this point is "shoulder well," describing the seemingly endless depth of this powerful point. Gallbladder 21 is another ultra-powerful acupressure point that can induce labor if pressed just right, driving energy down to your feet, dropping your blood pressure, and helping release your pelvic floor. It reduces adrenaline almost immediately, inviting oxytocin to inspire those big, efficient contractions that mama needs to birth her baby. Also:

it feels great!

Have mama seated on a birth ball or chair.

Stand behind her and lean forward so that your elbows are on acupressure point Gallbladder 21.

Begin with gentle, direct downward pressure and increase with mama's guidance until you reach her desired pressure. Release at her request.

Expert Tip: As the support person, use different areas of your elbow and forearm to change the pressure on this point.

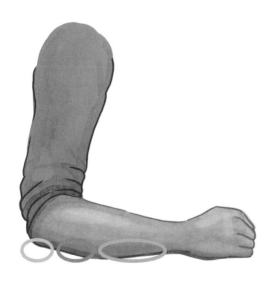

Intense   Medium   Mild

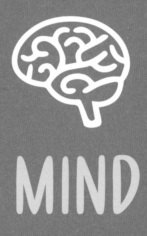

MIND

I've saved the best for last! If trained and treated kindly, mama's mind will be your greatest tool in labor. The mind is the key to our experiences; think of it as the lens that shapes reality. When we add a filter, things look different—sometimes brighter, sometimes darker. In this section, you will learn how to use the all-powerful mind to impact mama's physical experience.

It's the support partner's job to help focus mama's mind on the positive, quelling her concerns and reassuring her that she is prepared and capable of the task at hand. When you have some simple, familiar words, they come naturally and empower mama's confidence.

Practiced imagery scripts can dull mama's perception of pain, increasing pleasure and ultimately carrying her for hours. The pain management research on guided visualizations and hypnotherapy is so exciting, and birth educators have long been successfully utilizing these tools in labor. You'll find two examples of imagery scripts in the coming pages along with explanations of their indicated use.

Words of encouragement, known as affirmations, are always welcome *unless they aren't*, and then the best medicine is your silence and presence. Just be there and try mama's favorite SUPPORT, MOVE, and MASSAGE techniques. Stay open to her feedback, and mama will let you know what she needs and wants as labor runs its course.

Remember to layer your techniques. The mind is mama's central processor; it's the computer that's receiving information from the body and translating it into a feeling. Pain and pleasure signals are communicated from the body to the brain through wiring that we call nerves. You can interrupt the pain communication in two ways: peripherally at the nerves through massage, or centrally through the mind. For best results, layer MASSAGE and MIND!

Affirmations

In case you haven't gathered thus far: Labor can be long, and your loving support is absolutely crucial for the well-being of both mama and baby. Many of the MIND techniques are simple words of encouragement, often called affirmations.

The powerful hormones that govern birth also create a course of mental hurdles: Most women will experience various crises of confidence, waves of fear, and periods of exhaustion throughout labor. Affirming words will be the most helpful thing for her to hear. Read on for a variety of affirmations addressing the most common mental hurdles in labor.

Fear It's virtually impossible to describe the sensations of labor, not because they're so bad, but because they're so unique. The only time we experience the uterus doing its strong muscular work is in labor, and some women become scared that the contractions are too strong, or that something must be wrong for labor to feel as it does. These are common and normal feelings, and it's important to reassure her that her body is built for this intense process. Remind her that she is safe.

Crisis of Confidence How do you deeply know that you can give birth before you actually do it? Most of us don't. Most of us go through labor with some mix of disbelief and faith. There will be points in labor when this unfathomable feat feels impossible, and mama will usually vocalize this by saying, "I can't do this." Or labor will stall because her trust in her own abilities is going down and her oxytocin is going down with it. Your job is to support her with words of total support and belief in her abilities. Don't overthink it; just say it like you mean it.

Exhaustion The sedating impact of labor's natural hormones, and any narcotics used for pain medication, will make mama feel extremely tired, sometimes weak, and lightheaded. In an unmedicated labor, it's helpful to understand that drowsiness is the body's way of reducing the intensity of labor. When she's feeling too exhausted to go on, it's helpful to remind mama that she is strong, powerful, capable, and incredible!

Expert Tip:

You can repeat the same affirmations throughout labor; they won't get old.

Layer your support! You can use affirmations while you are using the SUPPORT, MOVE, and MASSAGE techniques

Perfect Birth

Women in labor are physically working very hard, and they may also be self-conscious while they are sweating and making noises usually reserved for the bedroom or the bathroom.

When she thinks she can't
stand any more, say:

" You are birthing your baby perfectly. This is very hard work, but you are birthing your baby perfectly. "

Trust

It's normal for a woman in labor to get nervous—scared even—and start to doubt her body's ability to give birth; it's a daunting task.

You can encourage her confidence by reminding her that her body knows how to give birth and that she is already doing such a good job. She trusts you, and she will appreciate your belief in her abilities.

Quietly say:

" **Trust this process. Your body knows how to give birth. You're doing so well.** "

Expert Tip: Keep it light! Practicing affirmations before labor can feel really cheesy. Don't take yourself too seriously. Simply do your best to internalize the words and explore how they make you feel. Just becoming familiar with the words will help them flow more naturally in labor.

MIND

Birth Story

My biggest fear all through pregnancy was labor.
Honestly, I really didn't trust that my body would work
with me, especially after being nauseous literally my entire
pregnancy. It was crucial for me to learn about birth, to hear
positive birth stories, and to really internalize that my body
is capable of birthing and my baby is capable of being
born—we grew together and we will birth together. I had to
trust in the process in order to get through labor.

Makeesha C.

Hospital   27 Hours   Nitrous Gas

Goddess

When mama is feeling anxious about the intensity of the contractions, or her body's ability to complete the job of labor, remind her that her body is capable and strong.

Quietly say:

" Look how well your body knows how to do this. You are a goddess. "

ACTIVITY
Courage

When I am feeling scared, I want you to say

_____

_____

_____

MIND

Perfect

Help build the laboring woman's confidence by telling her how well she is doing.

At the height of a contraction, say:

" That's perfect; that's wonderful. This is such hard work. You are wonderful! "

Beautiful

Help mama feel empowered and radiant by quietly saying:

" You are beautiful. You are glowing. You are so beautiful. "

ACTIVITY
Self-Assurance

Birth is all about mama's belief in herself.

Mama, think of yourself in the brightest, kindest light and share your positive adjectives:

"I believe I am . . ."

MIND

Remember: You will reduce mama's adrenaline and increase her oxytocin by reminding her that you're there for her, whatever she needs. This will build trust.

$$Trust = Oxytocin$$

$$Fear = Adrenaline$$

Most women will have moments in labor when they feel deeply alone, no matter how many people are in the room. It's easy to feel sorry for yourself during labor when you realize that you are the only one who can get this big job done.

But mama is **not** alone.

You are her cheering squad, hydration station, pit crew, massage therapist, labor coach, aromatherapist, and number one fan all rolled into one. Her medical team is available for safety support, and you are all on her team.

Support

Quietly say:

"I am here for you;
we are here for you.
You are doing such a
good job."

You Can Do It

Nearly every woman in labor will have a crisis of confidence, a moment when she is convinced that she can't go on.

When she thinks she can't stand any more, say:

" You can do this! Look at how far you've come! You are doing this. "

It's your job to encourage her and let her know how well she's doing when she thinks she can't stand any more.

With your encouraging words, you will help her know that she is strong and capable.

114

ACTIVITY
Confidence

When I'm worried that I can't do it, I want you to say

_____

_____

_____

_____

_____

MIND

Good Work

The continuous work of labor can be frustrating, and it is your job as labor support partner to keep mama's spirits high so she has the energy for the marathon.

*When she's working through
a contraction, slowly say:*

" That's right, just like that—
good work, just like that. "

Giving her positive feedback about her efforts will be appreciated, whether she lets you know that in the moment or not. Your words will help quell her anxiety that she may not be "doing it right."

Wonderful Job

In the midst of a long labor, it can be easy to forget what you're working toward: the birth of a baby. With every contraction, birth can feel more abstract and further away.

When things get tough for her, say:

"You are doing such a wonderful job; you get closer with each contraction. You are doing a wonderful job!"

Help your laboring partner keep her eye on the prize by reminding her of the purpose of these contractions: to open the cervix and bring her baby closer to birth.

Strong

The sedating impact of labor's natural hormones, and any narcotics used for pain medication, will make mama feel extremely tired and even weak. Additionally, it's normal for women to shake or shiver at different points in labor due to the healthy, normal labor hormones. The fatigue and the shaking can be alarming and even scary for some women.

Reflect her strength back to her by reminding her how strong she is and that you know she can do it.

Quietly say:

"
"You can do this; you are so strong. You can do this."
"

ACTIVITY
Strength

When I'm so exhausted that I want to give up,
I want you to say

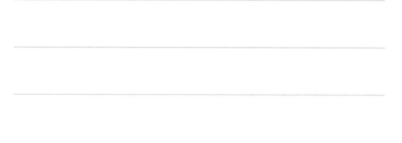

_____

_____

_____

_____

_____

Guided Imagery

Slowly read this script with a very calm, quiet voice:

"Slowly inhale through your nose and release it completely through your mouth.

"Feel the air move in and out, like an ocean breeze. Smell the salty ocean air, feel the ocean breeze on your face.

"Listen to the waves rolling in against the sand. Hear the soft roar of each wave rolling in, splashing onto the sand.

"Walk to the water; feel the wet sand in between your toes and under your feet with each step. Now, water is lapping onto your toes, your feet, your ankles.

"The breeze is cool against your face. The ocean water feels refreshing on your feet. Your body is completely relaxed as you feel the waves and the breeze on your skin.

"Stay with this feeling of relaxation as you continue to breathe through each wave, in and out."

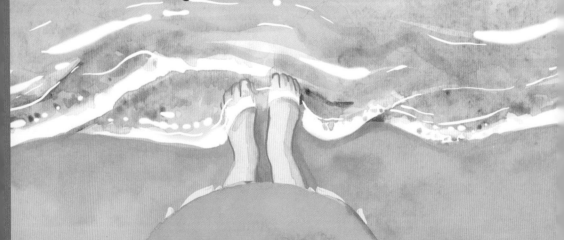

Guided imagery uses the mind-body connection to access an alternate state of being. Pain management research has shown us that envisioning a relaxing, beautiful scene will prompt your body to react as if it's been transported there. For example, if you're on a long walk through a hot desert, imagining that you're in a cold environment will help you cope with the hot temperature.

In the case of childbirth, our goal is to regulate blood pressure, reduce adrenaline, and increase oxytocin by inviting the mind to a comfortable, peaceful place. When you help mama envision this place, her mind is calmed and her body follows by releasing pleasure hormones. These hormones are the on-switch for labor. If a woman imagines she is in a comfortable, relaxing environment while she is in labor, she can better handle the intensity of each contraction.

Using the *Guided Imagery* script, talk mama through an ocean experience. Everyone's happy place is unique, so find out what mama's most relaxing scenario is. Is she on a mountain top? Floating on a lake? Hiking in the forest? Then craft a script just for her!

Hypnosis

"Slowly inhale through your nose, taking a deep breath in all the way to your belly, and release it completely through your mouth.

"Listen to the sound of my voice, and only the sound of my voice, and let your body relax, relax around each contraction.

"Relax so deeply that you melt into air. Let your body become light, let your body become as light as air, and every time you hear my voice you let yourself become much lighter.

"Imagine you are so light, so relaxed, that you are floating on a cloud. The cloud mist is the perfect temperature.

"Inhale... relax... exhale... relax... light as air... floating... You are as light as the cloud."

Repeat the script as many times as mama wants you to.

Hypnosis is a relaxation tool that can be extremely soothing in labor. It's *not* someone else controlling mama's mind; it's a tool to help her focus her mind and control her body's responsiveness to your supportive prompts.

Used therapeutically as a pain management tool, hypnosis reduces the perception of pain and associated anxiety. Rigorous research shows that hypnotherapy can be deeply effective for pain management, reducing the use of pain medication in a variety of scenarios including surgery.

Hypnosis is most effective when practiced regularly (at least 2 or 3 times a week) for a couple of months prior to labor. Practicing hypnosis will train the brain to drive out distractions, increasing mama's concentration and her receptivity to the suggestions of the speaker.

The relaxation script on the facing page is just one example of many, but a quick dive into the internet will show you a variety of programs that teach hypnosis for childbirth. We've included our favorites in the Resources section on page 142.

"A woman in birth is at once her most powerful, and most vulnerable. But any woman who has birthed unhindered understands that we are stronger than we know."

Marcie Macari

ACTIVITY
This or That, Take 2

Retake the test after you've practiced these strategies in preparation for labor. Revisit page 48 to see if any of your preferences have changed.

Hot	Cold
Shower	Bath
Sitting	Standing
Deep massage	Light touch
Chatting	Silence
Upbeat music	Relaxing music
Lots of people around	Very few people around
Water	Fruit juice
Self-guided	Guided by support person

Bonus activity: *Look back at this page after birth to see if your preferences were the same in labor!*

Common Hurdles & Suggested Techniques

Posterior Baby

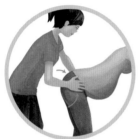 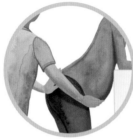 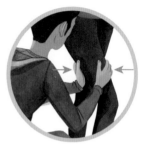

Double Hip Sweeze, p. 84   *Back & Belly Hold, p. 83*   *Shake the Tree, p. 90*

Back Labor

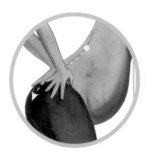 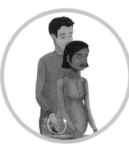 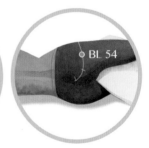

Lower Back Stroke, p. 94   *Belly Dance, p. 93*   *Tailbone Press, p. 86*

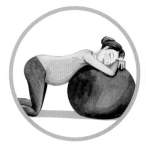

Lean on Ball, p. 69

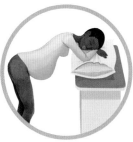

Lean on Counter p. 60

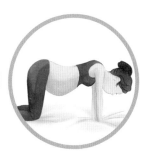

All Fours, p. 59

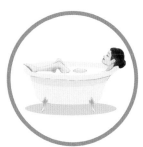

Bath, p. 38

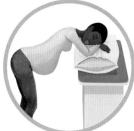

Lean on Counter, p. 60

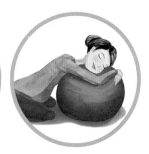

Relaxed Crouch, p. 68

Hip Pain

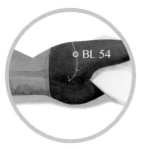

Bum Press, p. 97

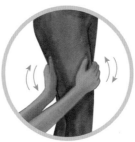

Shake the Tree, p. 90

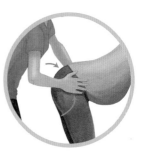

Double Hip Squeeze, p. 84

Stalled Labor

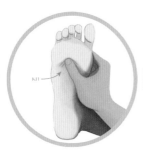

Foot Press, p. 98

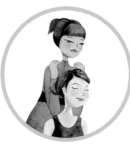

Shoulder Press, p. 100

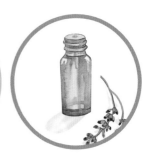

Aromatherapy, p. 29

Slow Dilation

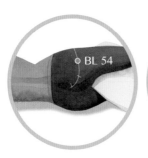

Bum Press, p. 97

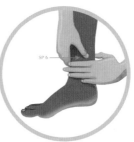

Ankle Press, p. 99

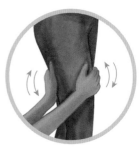

Shake the Tree, p. 90

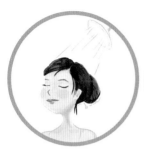

Shower, p. 39

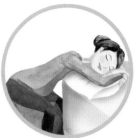

Ball & Bed, p. 66

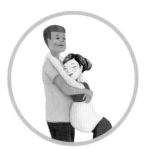

Slow Dance, p. 55

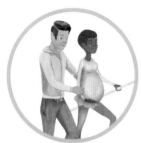

Walk, p. 56

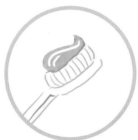

Brush Teeth, p. 57

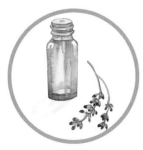

Aromatherapy, p. 29

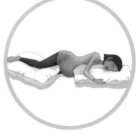

Side Lying, p. 70

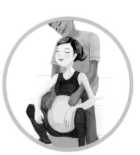

Squat p. 74

Epidural

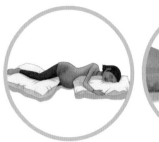 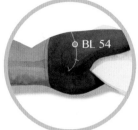 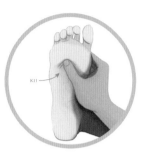

Side Lying, p. 70   *Bum Press, p. 97*   *Foot Press, p. 98*

Anxiety

 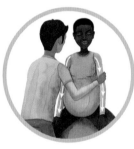 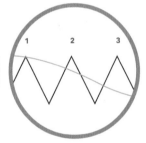

Lighting, p. 27   *Arm Stroke p. 89*   *Breath Pattern, p. 45*

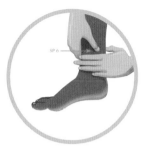

Ankle Press, p. 99

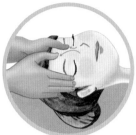

Third Eye Stroke p. 92

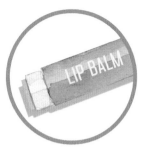

Lip Balm, p. 33

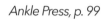

Trust
this process.
Your body knows
how to give birth.

Trust, p. 107

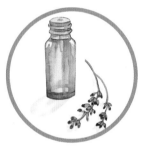

Aromatherapy, p. 29

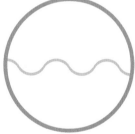

Groaning, p. 46

Layering Sequences

A few of our favorite combinations for ultimate support

Pre-Labor

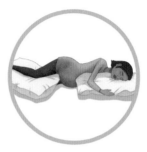
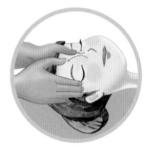

Lighting, p. 27   *Side Lying, p. 70*   *Third Eye Stroke, p. 92*

Early Labor

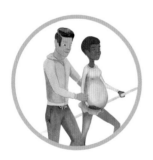
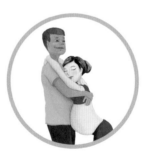
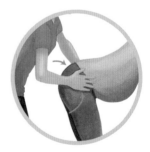

Walk, p. 56   *Slow Dance, p. 55*   *Double Hip Squeeze, p. 84*

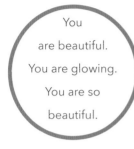

You are beautiful. You are glowing. You are so beautiful.

Beautiful, p. 110

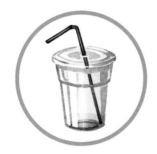

Hydration, p. 22

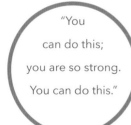

"You can do this; you are so strong. You can do this."

Strong, p. 118

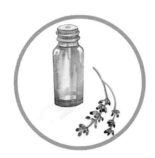

Aromatherapy, p. 29

Active Labor

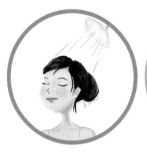
Shower, p. 39

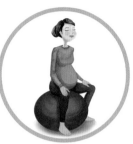
Ball Sit p. 64

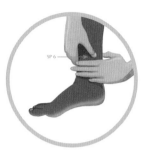
Ankle Press, p. 99

Active Labor

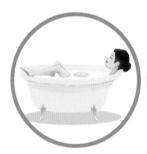
Bath, p. 38

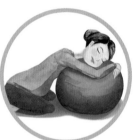
Relaxed Crouch, p. 68

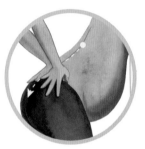
Lower Back Stroke, p. 94

Transition

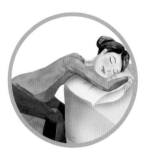
Ball & Bed, p. 66

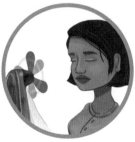
Fan, p. 35

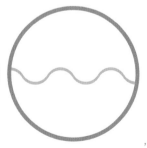
Groaning, p. 46

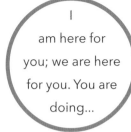

I am here for you; we are here for you. You are doing...

Support, p. 113

Slowly take a big breath deep into your belly, then let it go...

Cleansing Breath, p. 43

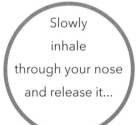

Slowly inhale through your nose and release it...

Guided Imagery, p. 120

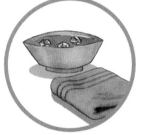

Wash Cloth, p.36

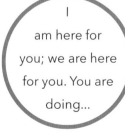

I am here for you; we are here for you. You are doing...

Support, p. 113

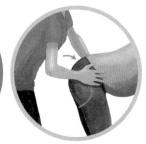

Double Hip Squeeze, p. 84

What Is a Doula?

A doula is your cheerleader for childbirth, your teacher, your advocate, your constant companion, and your physical support.

Your doula is trained in comfort techniques for labor, but she is not a medical professional and will not check your dilation or your baby's heart tones. A doula is not a midwife or a nurse.

In pregnancy a doula will teach you about labor and birth, helping you decipher your preferences in detail. They are a shoulder to lean on, an educated ear to listen, and a wealth of resources.

In early labor, your doula comes to your home to soothe you before it's time to go to your place of birth, if you're going to a birth center or hospital. They are there to support you as well as your partner, and can help make the transition to your place of birth smoother.

In the hospital or birth center, your doula is there to help you interpret the medical language and make decisions about your care. She will use tried-and-true techniques to help you navigate your labor journey. Most importantly, her expert care will be a constant throughout your labor while the birth center or hospital staff changes.

Your doula is there to support you and your partner, so you're both feeling confident and capable. If you're birthing without a partner present, your doula can be your primary support.

The right doula is different for every person and has little to do with how many births the doula has attended. Like all of birth, the most important factor is chemistry and comfort. Your personalities have to blend easily so you're all comfortable.

You need to trust your doula so that you feel safe in her care. Her primary job is reducing your adrenaline, increasing your oxytocin, and helping labor flow. Research shows that familiar birth support– a doula's specialty–reduces the need for pain medication and the likelihood of a caesarian birth, so use this doula interview guide as a start on your journey.

Why Hire a Doula?

- **less likely** to need Pitocin

- **less likely** to have a cesarean birth

- **less likely** to use any pain medication

- **more likely** to rate their childbirth experience positively

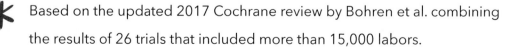

Based on the updated 2017 Cochrane review by Bohren et al. combining the results of 26 trials that included more than 15,000 labors.

Doula Questionnaire

- What are your fees?

- Why did you become a doula and what do you love about being a doula?

- How many births have you attended?

- Are you certified?

- What kind of training do you have?

- Have you attended births at my hospital or birth center? Or, if you are planning a home birth: Have you attended home births before?

- What's a challenging situation you've faced at a birth and how did you handle it?

- What are your core philosophies about birth?

- How do you feel about pain medication in labor?

- How would you describe your style of doula support?

- How do you help moms with fear?

- How do you help moms with pain?

- How will you support my partner to best support me?

- How do you work with the medical team?

- How many prenatal visits are included in your birth package?

- How many postpartum visits are included in your birth package?

- Will you come to my house in early labor or will you meet me at my place of birth?

- Do you stay for the entire labor and birth?

- Are you experienced and trained in helping with breastfeeding?

- How many weeks are you on call for my estimated due date?

- Do you have back-up support in case you're not available when I go into labor?

- How does your contract handle a change in birth plans if we no longer need labor support?

- Do you have client references I can check?

Birth Packing List

Labor Supplies:

♥ This book!

♥ *The Birth Deck*

♥ Favorite lip balm

♥ Electric fan

♥ Aromatherapy oils

♥ Favorite mints

♥ Large water bottle with straw

♥ Electric candles

♥ Super soft washcloth for cooling the face

♥ Bluetooth speaker and charger for music

♥ Snacks for mama—favorite energy bar cut into small pieces for easy snacking

♥ Snacks for support partner

♥ Gift for the hospital staff—chocolate always works

The Important Stuff:

♥ Phone and charger

♥ Driver's license, insurance card

♥ Hospital or birth center paperwork

Sundries:

- Essential toiletries:

    Toothbrush

    Toothpaste

    Deodorant

    Hair ties

    Lotion

    Lip balm

- Eyeglasses

- Baby journal and pen

- Slippers

For Mama*:

- Comfortable labor dress

- Warm robe

- Soft pajamas

- Loose pants for daytime

- Nursing pads

- Nursing bra or tank x 2

- Comfortable clothes for your journey home

For Baby:

- Swaddle blankets x 2

- Going-home outfit that will allow car seat to buckle

- Baby booties

- Car seat

✳ Do not bring anything you cherish; birth can be messy.

Resources

Pregnancy and Birth Education

BREECH OR POSTERIOR BABY
Spinning Babies   https://spinningbabies.com/

BIRTH EDUCATION
Pushing Power by Chantal Traub   www.chantaltraub.com/events
Mindful Birthing by Nancy Bardacke (New York: HarperOne, 2012)

HYPNOSIS FOR CHILDBIRTH
HypnoBirthing International   https://us.hypnobirthing.com/
Hypnobabies   https://www.hypnobabies.com/

DOULA DIRECTORY
Doula Match   https://doulamatch.net/

HOME BIRTH RESOURCES
Spiritual Midwifery by Ina May Gaskin (Summertown, TN: Book Publishing Company, 1975)
North American Registry of Midwives   http://narm.org/

Postpartum Preparation

POSTPARTUM MOOD DISORDERS
The Seleni Institute   http://www.seleni.org/

POSTPARTUM MEAL TRAIN PLANNING
MealTrain.com   https://www.mealtrain.com/

LACTATION SUPPORT
Boober   https://getboober.com/
Pacify   https://www.pacify.com/
La Leche League   https://www.llli.org/
Silverette Cups   https://www.silveretteusa.com/

BIRTH STORY PROCESSING
The Birth Journal   https://thebirthjournal.com/

Dear Mama,

When you look back at your labor, your sense of satisfaction will come from feeling that you were heard, that your needs were met, and that you were truly supported in your process. Research tells us that these factors matter more than what materially transpires during your labor—isn't that wild? Mind over matter. Vaginal birth, belly birth (C-section), long labor, short labor—if you were lovingly cared for, they can all be equally satisfying. Remember this as you prepare, as your set your vision. This work you and your support partner are doing right now is already making your future birth better.

Support Partner,

Exceptional support can come from anyone: friends, family, boyfriends, girlfriends, spouses, and doulas. You have the power to make mama's birth beautiful and fulfilling just by being present and adaptable. Learning about labor and birth is the most important thing you can do to support her in this exciting moment. The time and effort you're investing just by reading this book shows her you care, that you're listening to her needs and working to meet them. Your primary job is helping mama trust in herself, in her baby, and in her body. Your calm presence, confident voice, and gentle hands will be enough.

I am thinking of you both, and I know that you've got this!

With love,

Sara

About the Contributors

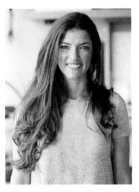

The founder of Glow Birth & Body, Sara Lyon brings her rich experience as a doula, childbirth educator, prenatal massage therapist, and mother to readers of *You've Got This*. An alumna of the University of Michigan and Australia's Endeavour College of Natural Medicine, Sara's career has focused on improving perinatal experiences and outcomes. Her publications, *The Birth Deck* and *You've Got This*, are extensions of Sara's effort to bring effective birth support into more hands. Sara and her family split their time between bustling New York City and the beautiful San Francisco Bay Area.

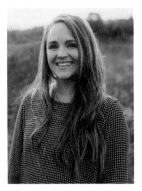

Brittany Mash, the illustrator and graphic designer of *You've Got This*, uses her background in neuroscience and medical illustration to create helpful and informative imagery for expectant mothers and their birth partners. Brittany, her husband, and her son live in mid-Michigan and enjoy spending their time traveling, hiking, and trying new coffee shops.